I0774092

ROSIE SANTOS

Hormone Hijinks

A Guide to Perimenopause and Menopause

This book was professionally typeset on Reedsy.
Find out more at reedsy.com

Contents

1

Introduction

The "M" word. When I was a kid, it was what all the older women, grandmas, great-grands, aunties, and sometimes men claimed when there was something physical happening to an "older" woman. That's all I could make of it. No other explanation. Fast forward 30 years later and I'm still in that place where **m e n o p a u s e** is what old ladies go through.

Today, I want to challenge all your understanding, experience, feelings, and outlook by sharing the facts about perimenopause and menopause. First, I will define both perimenopause and menopause, why it's all happening, and what it means. I will also outline the "menopause era" with you in phases and share all the specifics of each phase. Next, I will share the physiology of the adrenal system and how your hormones are major players during perimenopause and menopause. These will form the reasoning behind all the "hijinks" expressed as symptoms that span over years and are unique to each woman, however, there are common symptoms to look out for.

Lastly, so we're not left in the dark with the "M" word and feeling lost about this time in our lives, we are grateful there are treatments and ways to alleviate the negative experience of going through perimenopause and menopause. I'm writing this book for my daughters and nieces and my future granddaughters and my friends' daughters and their future granddaughters. My encouragement to you is to take a deep breath knowing you're not alone. This is real, there are ways to help you, and it's all very normal. So, dive into this resource with your sleep-deprived eyes, chubby middle, and cloudy brain. I'll make it simple for you because I'm right there with you.

My Journey: Is this it?

I never thought it would happen this soon. Is it happening? Or was it happening years ago and I didn't realize it? I had 4 kids in 8 years. My lady parts served me well. Fertile lady parts and I will never take that for granted. But these very lady parts are now betraying me.

If I were to understand what I'm going through right now, which is perimenopause, I want to go further back and share how my hormones were functioning throughout my life. Not only the actual physical way my hormones were manifesting but really HOW I FELT in every girl era of my life. The first time I would ever acknowledge my womanhood would be in 5th grade. The budding breasts and ugh..the onset of my first period at the age of 10. Mom said this is when she started hers. It was what we go through as women for a greater part of our lives. I hated it. It was gross. It felt gross and my body hurt. I didn't want it. The bleeding and changing of the pad. Contemplating whether to use a tampon. Are my friends going through this too? Will people KNOW I have it? And, what...every month! The torture. I didn't ask for this. It's not fair. This was the first time I felt anxiety and depression. I was coming to terms that this is what I had to go through. But then, on the upside, now I'm feeling attracted to boys. Like a real physical and emotional connection. My body would feel tingly whenever I thought a boy liked me. If you were to ask my mom and friends, my high-hormonal era was in full force from age 12 to 21. And it was true. Uncontrollable. The ups and downs of emotion. One day I'm elated, the next day I'm down in the dumps. Like the world was ending. Then it was the crushes and acting impulsively to sexual attraction. My body was betraying me in a weird but fun way.

Heading into my 20s, all of those same feelings of strong physical attraction to men, the highs and lows of emotion were a bit more tamed. More controlled and less intense. This is where I felt I was cruising in my womanhood. My mind was clear and I was focused on what I wanted in life: a career, a marriage, and kids. It was all there in front of me. Nothing can stand in my way. That's the best part of the 20s. You do feel you can do anything you want. I married the love of my life at 26 and the following year I got pregnant.

Here we go again with the hormones. Even though the physical part of it was obvious because I was growing a human inside of me, the emotional part was haywire at times. I was anxious, excited, lonely, and angry. It was all the above, any day, all days, all the time. Then after the pregnancy, it felt like confusion. I wanted to feel elation and love for my new baby but I felt like the world was against me and I was helpless and alone and there was nothing good left for me. SO CONFUSING. SO lonely. So sad. I knew little about postpartum depression and I didn't get treatment so it was a journey of learning how to strengthen my heart and mind and knowing how to ask for support. This all happened 4 times to me. But with each time, progressively easier and harder at the same time. If you make me tell you how I can't. It's done and it was a blur. All I know is the whirlwind of having kids in itself is survival.

Fast forward to after my last child. I started having parts of me fail. My hair started thinning and my skin would have unexplained rashes. Weight loss got harder. Instead of the lean 120 lbs I was in my 20s, now I stayed at a constant 130 lbs and I couldn't shed no matter what I did. And this became worse and worse as I went into my 40s. More weight, less hair, bad skin, more anxiety, less libido, more sadness and depression. Is this it? I tried to remember when my mom started menopause and when she first mentioned it. I was in high school and then in college when she started acting on it. It was like war. Her crash diets and exercise obsession. Lots of walking and swimming. She even had a small stroke in her mid-50s. That was scary. And not to mention all the gaslighting my family was giving her to her complaints of body pain, dizziness, brain fog. She seemed like a hypochondriac for a good 10 years. Then it stopped. Even though the doctor gave her the diagnosis of lupus, coined as the catchall diagnosis when they couldn't explain what was wrong.

Here I am in the same place as my Mom in her mid-40s. I'm feeling like I'm not myself anymore and I don't know why. My body is betraying me.

2

The Beginning of a New Era: Perimenopause and Menopause

Welcome to the beginning of a new era in your life! Perimenopause and menopause are often seen as daunting transitions, but they are also times of significant personal growth and transformation. Let's embark on this journey with a spirit of curiosity and optimism as we delve into what these stages mean, how they differ, and what you can expect.

What is Perimenopause?

Perimenopause, often referred to as the "menopausal transition," is the period leading up to menopause. During this time, your body begins to make the natural transition toward permanent infertility, marking the end of your reproductive years. But don't let the term "end" mislead you—this is also a beginning, a time to embrace new opportunities for health, wellness, and self-discovery.

Perimenopause can start as early as your mid-30s but typically begins in your 40s. It's characterized by a series of hormonal changes as your ovaries gradually produce less estrogen and progesterone, the hormones that regulate menstruation. This phase can last anywhere from a few months to several years, with the average duration being around four years. However, for some women, it can extend up to ten years.

Distinction Between Perimenopause and Menopause

It's essential to understand the distinction between perimenopause and menopause, as these terms are often used interchangeably but refer to different stages of this life transition.

Perimenopause is the transition phase before menopause. It is marked by fluctuating hormone levels, which lead to various physical and emotional symptoms. During perimenopause, you might still have menstrual periods, although they can become irregular—shorter, longer, lighter, or heavier.

Menopause, on the other hand, is defined as the point in time when you have not had a menstrual period for 12 consecutive months. This marks the official end of your menstrual cycle. The average age of menopause in women in the United States is 51, but it can occur in your 40s or 50s. Once you reach menopause, your body produces very low levels of the reproductive hormones estrogen and progesterone.

In summary, perimenopause is the journey, and menopause is the destination. But remember, the journey itself is rich with experiences that can lead to greater self-awareness and well-being.

Typical Age Range and Duration of Perimenopause

Perimenopause typically begins in a woman's 40s, but some women may start experiencing changes as early as their mid-30s. The exact age at which perimenopause starts can vary widely from person to person, influenced by factors such as genetics, lifestyle, and overall health.

The duration of perimenopause is also variable. On average, it lasts about four years, but it can be as short as a few months or extend up to a decade. This variability is entirely normal, and there's no "one-size-fits-all" timeline. Some women may breeze through this phase with minimal discomfort, while others might experience a more prolonged and symptomatic transition.

Embracing the Changes

While the thought of hormonal fluctuations might seem overwhelming, it's important to approach perimenopause with a positive mindset. This era is not just about endings but about new beginnings. It's a time to prioritize your health, reflect on your achievements, and set new goals for the future.

Many women find that perimenopause is an opportunity to re-evaluate their lifestyles and make beneficial changes.

Embracing a New Chapter: Understanding Menopause

Welcome to the next chapter of your journey—menopause! This stage marks a significant milestone in every woman's life, representing the end of menstruation and the beginning of a new era of freedom and self-discovery. Let's explore what menopause means, its biological significance, the average age of onset, and the factors that influence its timing. We'll approach this topic with an upbeat and hopeful tone, celebrating the possibilities and opportunities that menopause brings.

What is Menopause?

Menopause is defined as the point in time when a woman has not experienced a menstrual period for 12 consecutive months. This natural biological process marks the end of reproductive years, as the ovaries cease producing eggs and the levels of estrogen and progesterone—the hormones responsible for regulating menstruation—significantly decrease.

While menopause is often viewed as an end, it is also a beginning. It signifies a transition into a new phase of life where you can embrace changes, prioritize your well-being, and focus on personal growth. Menopause is not an illness but a natural stage of aging, and it can be a time of empowerment and renewal.

Biological Significance of Menopause

The biological significance of menopause lies in its role as a natural evolutionary process. Here are some key aspects of its biological importance:

1. End of Reproductive Function:

Menopause marks the end of a woman's reproductive capabilities. This transition signifies that the ovaries no longer release eggs, and menstruation ceases. While this may seem like a significant change, it is a natural progression that allows the body to shift its focus from reproduction to other vital functions.

2. Hormonal Adjustments:

The decline in estrogen and progesterone levels during menopause leads to various physiological adjustments. These hormonal changes affect multiple systems in the body, including the cardiovascular system, bones, skin, and metabolism. Understanding these changes can help women manage symptoms and maintain overall health.

3. Evolutionary Perspective:

From an evolutionary standpoint, menopause may have developed as a way to ensure that older women could invest their time and resources in the survival and well-being of their offspring and grandchildren, rather than continuing to bear children. This perspective highlights the value of wisdom and experience that postmenopausal women bring to their families and communities.

The Average Age of Menopause

The average age of menopause for women in the United States is 51 years, but the timing can vary widely. Most women experience menopause between the ages of 45 and 55. However, some women may enter menopause as early as their 30s or as late as their 60s.

The age at which menopause occurs is influenced by various factors, including genetics, lifestyle, and overall health. It's important to remember that every woman's experience is unique, and there is no "right" or "wrong" age for menopause to occur.

Factors Influencing the Timing of Menopause

Several factors can influence the timing of menopause, and understanding these can provide insight into your own experience. Here are some key factors:

1. Genetics:

Your genetic makeup plays a significant role in determining the age at which you will reach menopause. If your mother or sisters experienced early or late menopause, you might follow a similar pattern. Family history is a strong indicator of menopausal timing.

2. Lifestyle Factors:

Lifestyle choices, such as smoking, diet, and physical activity, can impact the timing of menopause. For example, smoking has been shown to accelerate the onset of menopause by up to two years. On the other hand, a healthy diet and regular exercise can promote overall well-being and potentially influence the timing of menopause.

3. Medical Conditions and Treatments:

Certain medical conditions and treatments can affect menopausal timing. For instance, autoimmune diseases, thyroid disorders, and surgical removal of the ovaries (oophorectomy) can lead to earlier menopause. Additionally, cancer treatments like chemotherapy and radiation therapy can impact ovarian function and hasten menopause.

4. Reproductive History:

Your reproductive history, including the age at which you had your first period (menarche) and the number of pregnancies you've had, can also influence the timing of menopause. Some studies suggest that women who had their first period at an earlier age may experience menopause later.

5. Body Mass Index (BMI):

Body weight and fat distribution can impact estrogen levels in the body. Women with a higher BMI may have higher estrogen levels, potentially delaying the onset of menopause. Conversely, women with a lower BMI may experience menopause earlier.

The Phases of Perimenopause to Menopause

Transitioning from perimenopause to menopause is a significant journey marked by various phases, each with its own unique set of changes and milestones. Understanding these phases can help you navigate this period with greater ease and confidence. Let's explore the typical age range, key markers, and milestones of each phase in this journey.

Phase 1: Early Perimenopause
Typical Age Range:Late 30s to early 40s

Markers and Milestones:

1. **Irregular Periods:** The first noticeable sign of early perimenopause is changes in menstrual cycle regularity. Periods may become shorter, longer, heavier, or lighter.
2. **Hormonal Fluctuations:** Estrogen and progesterone levels begin to fluctuate, leading to symptoms such as mild hot flashes, night sweats, and mood swings.
3. **Fertility Changes:** Although it's still possible to conceive, fertility starts to decline during this phase.

During early perimenopause, these changes can be subtle and easily attributed to other factors like stress or lifestyle changes. It's essential to track your cycle and symptoms to recognize the onset of this phase.

Phase 2: Late Perimenopause
Typical Age Range: Mid to late 40s

Markers and Milestones:

1. **More Pronounced Cycle Changes**: Menstrual cycles become even more irregular, with longer gaps between periods or occasional skipped cycles.
2. **Intensified Symptoms:** Hot flashes, night sweats, mood swings, and sleep disturbances often become more pronounced and frequent.
3. **Vaginal and Urinary Changes:** Decreased estrogen levels

can lead to vaginal dryness, discomfort during intercourse, and urinary incontinence or infections.

Late perimenopause is characterized by more significant hormonal shifts and symptoms that can impact daily life. It's a time to focus on managing symptoms and maintaining overall health through diet, exercise, and stress reduction techniques.

Phase 3: Menopause
Typical Age Range: Early 50s (average age is 51)

Markers and Milestones:

1. **Final Menstrual Period**: Menopause is officially reached when you have gone 12 consecutive months without a menstrual period.
2. **End of Fertility**: Menopause marks the end of natural fertility, as the ovaries cease to release eggs.
3. **Stable Hormone Levels**: While hormone levels are lower than before, they stabilize, leading to a reduction in some perimenopausal symptoms.

The transition to menopause signifies the end of the menstrual cycle and reproductive years. This phase often brings relief from the unpredictability of perimenopausal symptoms, although some symptoms like hot flashes and night sweats may persist for a while.

Phase 4: Postmenopause
Typical Age Range: Beyond early 50s

Markers and Milestones:

1. **Symptom Management**: Many women find that symptoms gradually decrease in intensity, though some may continue to experience hot flashes and other symptoms for several years.
2. **Focus on Health**: Postmenopause is a critical time to focus on long-term health, particularly bone health, cardiovascular health, and maintaining a healthy weight.
3. **Embracing New Opportunities**: This phase offers the chance to embrace new hobbies, career opportunities, and personal growth without the concerns of menstruation or pregnancy.

Postmenopause is a period of stabilization and renewal. Women can enjoy the benefits of no longer dealing with menstrual cycles and can focus on enhancing their quality of life through proactive health measures and self-care.

Conclusion

The journey from perimenopause to menopause and beyond is marked by distinct phases, each with its challenges and milestones. By understanding these phases and their typical age ranges, you can better prepare for and navigate this natural transition. Embrace this journey with an open mind and a hopeful heart, knowing that each phase brings new opportunities for growth and self-discovery.

3

The Adrenal System and The Female Body

Understanding the intricate relationship between the adrenal system and the female body is crucial, especially during the phases of perimenopause and menopause. This chapter will provide an in-depth overview of the adrenal glands and their hormone functions, the connection between adrenal health and reproductive hormones, and the hormonal changes that occur during perimenopause and menopause. We will also explore how stress affects adrenal health and hormone balance and share effective techniques to manage stress for optimal well-being.

The Role of the Adrenal Glands

The adrenal glands are small, triangular-shaped glands located on top of each kidney. Despite their size, they play a significant role in regulating various bodily functions through the production of hormones. The adrenal glands consist of two main parts: the adrenal cortex and the adrenal medulla, each responsible for producing different types of hormones.

1. The Adrenal Cortex:

Glucocorticoids (e.g., cortisol): These hormones are essential for metabolism regulation, immune response, and stress management. Cortisol, often referred to as the "stress hormone," helps the body respond to stress and maintain homeostasis.

Mineralocorticoids (e.g., aldosterone):These hormones regulate sodium and potassium balance, and therefore, fluid balance and blood pressure.

Androgens: While primarily known as male hormones, androgens are also produced in small amounts by the adrenal glands in women and contribute to overall hormonal balance.

2. The Adrenal Medulla:

Catecholamines (e.g., adrenaline and noradrenaline): These hormones are involved in the body's fight-or-flight response, preparing the body to respond to stressful situations by increasing heart rate, blood pressure, and energy availability.

Hormonal Function and the Adrenal Glands

The adrenal glands are integral to maintaining hormonal balance in the body. They interact closely with other endocrine glands, such as the ovaries, to regulate a woman's reproductive system. This interaction is particularly significant during the phases of perimenopause and menopause.

1. Cortisol and Stress Response:

Cortisol helps the body respond to stress by increasing glucose levels for immediate energy and suppressing non-essential functions like digestion and immune response. Chronic stress can lead to prolonged elevated cortisol levels, which can negatively impact health.

2. Aldosterone and Blood Pressure Regulation:

Aldosterone helps regulate blood pressure by controlling the balance of sodium and potassium in the blood. The proper function of this hormone is essential for cardiovascular health.

3. Androgens and Hormonal Balance:

Although androgens are present in lower levels in women compared to men, they are crucial for libido, energy levels, and overall hormonal balance.

Adrenal Health and Reproductive Hormones

The health of the adrenal glands is closely connected to reproductive hormones such as estrogen and progesterone. This connection becomes especially important during the transitional phases of perimenopause and menopause.

1. Estrogen and Progesterone Balance:

Estrogen and progesterone are primary female reproductive hormones produced mainly by the ovaries. These hormones regulate the menstrual cycle, support pregnancy, and affect various other body functions, including bone density and cardiovascular health.

During the reproductive years, the ovaries are the primary source of these hormones. However, as women approach perimenopause, ovarian hormone production begins to fluctuate and eventually decline.

2. The Role of Adrenal Glands in Hormonal Balance:

As ovarian hormone production decreases, the adrenal glands play a supportive role in maintaining hormonal balance by producing small amounts of estrogen and progesterone precursors. Healthy adrenal function becomes vital for mitigating the effects of declining ovarian hormones.

Hormonal Changes During Perimenopause and Menopause

Perimenopause and menopause bring significant hormonal changes that impact the adrenal glands and overall health. Understanding these changes can help women navigate this transition more smoothly.

1. Perimenopause:

Hormonal Fluctuations: Perimenopause typically begins in a woman's 40s but can start as early as the mid-30s. During this phase, estrogen and progesterone levels fluctuate unpredictably, leading to irregular menstrual cycles and various symptoms such as hot flashes, mood swings, and sleep disturbances.

Adrenal Support: The adrenal glands help buffer these hormonal fluctuations by producing small amounts of estrogen and progesterone. However, if the adrenal glands are overworked or compromised due to chronic stress, this support may be insufficient, exacerbating perimenopausal symptoms.

2. Menopause:

Hormonal Decline: Menopause is defined as the absence of menstrual periods for 12 consecutive months, typically occurring around age 51. During menopause, the ovaries cease hormone production, leading to a significant decline in estrogen and progesterone levels.

Adrenal Compensation: Post-menopause, the adrenal glands continue to provide hormonal support, but their capacity to produce hormones is limited. Maintaining adrenal health is crucial to managing menopausal symptoms and supporting overall well-being.

Impact of Stress on Adrenal Health and Hormone Balance

Stress has a profound impact on the adrenal glands and overall hormonal balance. Chronic stress can lead to adrenal fatigue, affecting the production of cortisol and other hormones, which can exacerbate menopausal symptoms and affect overall health.

1. The Stress Response:

When the body perceives stress, the adrenal glands release cortisol and adrenaline to prepare for a fight-or-flight response.

This acute response is beneficial for short-term stress but becomes detrimental when stress is chronic.

Chronic stress keeps cortisol levels elevated, which can suppress immune function, increase inflammation, and disrupt other hormonal balances, including reproductive hormones.

2. Adrenal Fatigue:

Prolonged stress can lead to adrenal fatigue, a condition where the adrenal glands become overworked and unable to produce adequate levels of cortisol. Symptoms of adrenal fatigue include chronic fatigue, difficulty waking up, salt and sugar cravings, and decreased stress tolerance.

Adrenal fatigue can worsen menopausal symptoms, as the adrenal glands struggle to compensate for declining ovarian hormone production.

Techniques to Manage Stress and Support Adrenal Health

Managing stress is essential for maintaining adrenal health and hormonal balance, especially during perimenopause and menopause. Here are some effective techniques to help reduce stress and support overall well-being:

1. Regular Exercise:

Engaging in regular physical activity can help reduce stress levels and improve overall health. Activities such as yoga, walking, swimming, and strength training can enhance mood, improve sleep, and reduce anxiety.

2. Balanced Diet:

A nutritious diet rich in fruits, vegetables, lean proteins, and healthy fats supports adrenal health and hormone balance. Avoiding excessive caffeine, sugar, and processed foods can help maintain stable energy levels and reduce stress.

3. Mindfulness and Meditation:

Practices such as mindfulness meditation, deep breathing exercises, and progressive muscle relaxation can help reduce stress and promote a sense of calm. Regular mindfulness practice has been shown to lower cortisol levels and improve overall well-being.

4. Adequate Sleep:

Prioritizing good sleep hygiene is crucial for adrenal health and stress management. Aim for 7–9 hours of quality sleep per night by maintaining a consistent sleep schedule, creating a relaxing bedtime routine, and ensuring a comfortable sleep environment.

5. Social Support:

Building and maintaining strong social connections can provide emotional support and reduce feelings of isolation and stress. Engaging in social activities, joining support groups, and spending time with loved ones can enhance emotional well-being.

6. Time Management and Self-Care:

Effective time management and self-care practices can help reduce stress by ensuring a balance between work, family, and personal time. Setting realistic goals, taking regular breaks, and engaging in activities you enjoy can help maintain a healthy work-life balance.

7. Professional Support:

Seeking professional support from healthcare providers, therapists, or counselors can be beneficial in managing stress and adrenal health. Cognitive-behavioral therapy (CBT) and other therapeutic approaches can help develop effective coping strategies and improve overall mental health.

Conclusion

The adrenal system plays a vital role in regulating hormonal balance and supporting overall health, particularly during the transitional phases of perimenopause and menopause. Understanding the function of the adrenal glands and their interaction with reproductive hormones can help women navigate these changes more effectively. Managing stress is essential for maintaining adrenal health and ensuring a smoother transition through perimenopause and menopause. By incorporating stress-reducing techniques and prioritizing self-care, women can support their adrenal health, enhance their well-being, and embrace this new phase of life with confidence and optimism.

4

Navigating the Symptoms of Perimenopause and Menopause

Perimenopause and menopause are significant transitions in a woman's life, marked by a range of physical, emotional, and psychological symptoms. While these changes can be challenging, understanding and recognizing the symptoms can empower you to manage them effectively and maintain a positive outlook. In this chapter, we will explore the various symptoms associated with perimenopause and menopause, offering insights and encouragement to help you navigate this transformative time.

Symptoms of Perimenopause

Perimenopause is the transitional phase leading up to menopause, typically beginning in a woman's 40s but sometimes starting as early as the mid-30s. This phase is characterized by hormonal fluctuations that can lead to a variety of symptoms. Here are some common symptoms to look out for:

1. Irregular Periods:

One of the first signs of perimenopause is changes in menstrual cycle regularity. Periods may become shorter, longer, heavier, or lighter. You might also experience missed periods or spotting between cycles.

Tip: Keep a menstrual diary to track changes in your cycle. This information can help you and your healthcare provider understand your transition and manage symptoms effectively.

2. Hot Flashes and Night Sweats:

Hot flashes are sudden feelings of intense heat, often accompanied by sweating and a red, flushed face. Night sweats are similar but occur during sleep, potentially disrupting your rest.

Tip: Dress in layers, use a fan, and keep your bedroom cool at night. These simple adjustments can help manage hot flashes and night sweats, ensuring more comfortable days and restful nights.

3. Sleep Disturbances:

Many women experience difficulties with sleep during perimenopause, including trouble falling asleep, staying asleep, or waking up too early.

Tip: Establish a relaxing bedtime routine, avoid caffeine and electronics before bed, and create a comfortable sleep environment to improve sleep quality.

4. Mood Changes:

Hormonal fluctuations can lead to mood swings, irritability, anxiety, and even depression. These emotional changes can be challenging to manage.

Tip: Practice mindfulness, meditation, and deep breathing exercises to help regulate mood. Seeking support from friends, family, or a therapist can also provide valuable emotional relief.

5. Vaginal Dryness and Discomfort:

Decreased estrogen levels can cause vaginal dryness, itching, and discomfort during intercourse. This can lead to decreased libido and changes in sexual function.

Tip: Use water-based lubricants or vaginal moisturizers to alleviate dryness and discomfort. Communicate openly with your partner about these changes to maintain intimacy and connection.

6. Weight Gain and Changes in Body Composition:

Hormonal changes can lead to weight gain, especially around the abdomen. You might also notice changes in muscle mass and fat distribution.

Tip: Focus on a balanced diet rich in whole foods and engage in regular physical activity, including strength training, to maintain a healthy weight and body composition.

7. Cognitive Changes:

Some women experience memory lapses, difficulty concentrating, or what is often referred to as "brain fog."

Tip: Stay mentally active by engaging in puzzles, reading, and learning new skills. Regular exercise and a healthy diet can also support cognitive function.

Symptoms of Menopause

Menopause is defined as the point in time when a woman has not had a menstrual period for 12 consecutive months. This typically occurs around the age of 51 but can vary widely. The symptoms of menopause can overlap with those of perimenopause but may also bring new challenges.

1. Continuation of Hot Flashes and Night Sweats:

Hot flashes and night sweats may continue into menopause but often decrease in frequency and intensity over time.

Tip: Persist with strategies to manage these symptoms, and remember that they typically lessen as your body adjusts to new hormone levels.

2. Vaginal and Urinary Symptoms:

Vaginal dryness, itching, and discomfort may persist or worsen in menopause. You may also experience urinary incontinence or frequent urinary tract infections.

Tip: Continue using lubricants and moisturizers. Pelvic floor exercises (Kegels) can strengthen the muscles around the bladder and help with urinary symptoms.

3. Bone Density Loss:

The decline in estrogen levels can lead to decreased bone density, increasing the risk of osteoporosis and fractures.

Tip: Ensure adequate calcium and vitamin D intake, engage in weight-bearing exercises, and discuss bone density screening with your healthcare provider to maintain strong bones.

4. Changes in Sexual Function:

Decreased libido and changes in sexual response are common in menopause.

Tip: Explore new ways to enhance intimacy and pleasure. Open communication with your partner and seeking advice from a healthcare provider can help address sexual concerns.

5. Cardiovascular Health:

Post-menopausal women have an increased risk of cardiovascular disease due to changes in lipid profiles and blood pressure.

Tip: Adopt a heart-healthy lifestyle by eating a balanced diet, exercising regularly, managing stress, and avoiding smoking.

Emotional and Psychological Symptoms

The emotional and psychological impact of perimenopause and menopause can be profound, affecting mental health and overall well-being. Recognizing and addressing these symptoms is essential for maintaining a positive outlook during this transition.

1. Anxiety and Depression:

Hormonal changes can contribute to increased anxiety and depression. Feelings of sadness, hopelessness, and lack of interest in usual activities can be common.

Tip: Don't hesitate to seek help. Therapy, support groups, and medication can provide relief. Practicing self-compassion and engaging in activities that bring joy can also improve mood.

2. Mood Swings and Irritability:

Fluctuating hormone levels can lead to mood swings and irritability, making it challenging to maintain emotional stability.

Tip: Practice mindfulness and stress management techniques. Regular physical activity can also help stabilize mood by releasing endorphins.

3. Feelings of Loss and Identity Changes:

The transition through menopause can bring feelings of loss related to the end of fertility and changes in body image. Women may also experience shifts in their sense of identity and purpose.

Tip: View this phase as an opportunity for self-discovery and growth. Engage in new hobbies, pursue interests, and set new goals to redefine this stage of life positively.

4. Cognitive Challenges:

Memory lapses and difficulty concentrating can be frustrating and may impact daily functioning.

Tip: Keep your brain active with puzzles, reading, and learning new skills. Establish routines and use organizational tools to help manage cognitive changes.

5. Social and Relationship Dynamics:

Changes in mood, libido, and energy levels can affect relationships with partners, family, and friends.

Tip: Communicate openly with loved ones about what you're experiencing. Building a strong support network can provide emotional support and understanding.

Embracing the Transition with Positivity

Perimenopause and menopause are natural phases of life that every woman experiences. While the symptoms can be challenging, they also offer an opportunity for growth, self-care, and renewal. Here are some strategies to embrace this transition with positivity and hope:

1. Educate Yourself:

Knowledge is empowering. Understanding the changes happening in your body can alleviate anxiety and help you make informed decisions about your health.

Tip: Read books, attend workshops, and consult healthcare professionals to stay informed about perimenopause and menopause.

2. Prioritize Self-Care:

Make self-care a priority. Engage in activities that bring you joy and relaxation, whether it's yoga, meditation, gardening, or spending time with loved one

Tip: Taking care of yourself physically, emotionally, and mentally can enhance your overall well-being and help you navigate symptoms more effectively.

3. Stay Active:

Regular physical activity can help manage weight, improve mood, and support overall health.

Tip: Find activities you enjoy, such as walking, swimming, or dancing. Exercise not only benefits your body but also boosts your mental and emotional well-being.

4. Build a Support Network:

Connecting with other women going through similar experiences can provide valuable support and understanding.

Tip: Join support groups, both in-person and online, to share experiences and gain insights from others.

5. Focus on Nutrition:

A balanced diet rich in fruits, vegetables, lean proteins, and healthy fats can support hormonal balance and overall health.

Tip: Pay attention to your nutritional needs, and consider consulting a nutritionist for personalized advice.

6. Seek Professional Help:

If you experience severe symptoms or emotional distress, seek professional help. Healthcare providers, therapists, and counselors can offer guidance and treatment options.

Tip: Don't hesitate to reach out for support. Taking proactive steps to address symptoms can significantly improve your quality of life.

Conclusion

The journey through perimenopause and menopause is unique for every woman, marked by a variety of physical, emotional, and psychological symptoms. By understanding and recognizing these symptoms, you can take proactive steps to manage them effectively and maintain a positive outlook. Embrace this transition as an opportunity for growth and self-care, and remember that you are not alone—many women share your experiences and are here to support you. With knowledge,

self-care, and a supportive network, you can navigate perimenopause and menopause with confidence and optimism,
embracing this new chapter of life with grace and resilience.

5

Enhancing Quality of Life During Perimenopause and Menopause

Navigating through perimenopause and menopause can be a transformative journey. While these stages bring about various physical and emotional changes, numerous treatments and lifestyle adjustments can significantly enhance your quality of life. This chapter explores hormone therapy, natural and alternative therapies, lifestyle changes, and emotional and mental health support, offering a comprehensive approach to managing this transition with optimism and hope.

Hormone Therapy

Hormone therapy (HT) is a well-established treatment for alleviating menopausal symptoms. It involves supplementing the body with estrogen, or a combination of estrogen and progesterone, to balance hormone levels.

1. Estrogen Therapy (ET):

Purpose: Primarily used for women who have had a hysterectomy, as estrogen alone can increase the risk of endometrial cancer if the uterus is still present.

Benefits: ET effectively reduces hot flashes, night sweats, and vaginal dryness, and prevents bone loss.

2. Combination Therapy:

Purpose: For women who still have their uterus, a combination of estrogen and progesterone is prescribed to counteract the risk of endometrial cancer.

Benefits: Besides alleviating menopausal symptoms, it helps in maintaining bone density and reducing the risk of osteoporosis.

Considerations and Risks:

Hormone therapy is not suitable for everyone. Women with a history of breast cancer, blood clots, or liver disease, or those who are at high risk for these conditions may need to avoid HT.

Side effects can include bloating, breast tenderness, headaches, and mood changes. It is essential to discuss the risks and benefits with your healthcare provider to determine the best course of action.

Tip: If hormone therapy is appropriate for you, it can significantly improve your quality of life by alleviating many of the disruptive symptoms of menopause. Regular check-ups and open communication with your healthcare provider are crucial for monitoring your progress and adjusting treatment as needed.

Natural and Alternative Therapies

Many women seek natural and alternative therapies as a complement or alternative to hormone therapy. These treatments can provide relief from symptoms and support overall well-being.

1. Phytoestrogens:

Sources: Found in soy products, flaxseeds, and certain herbs like red clover.

Benefits: Phytoestrogens are plant-based compounds that mimic estrogen in the body and can help reduce hot flashes and improve vaginal health.

2. Herbal Supplements:

Black Cohosh: Often used to alleviate hot flashes and night sweats.

Evening Primrose Oil: Can help with breast tenderness and mood swings.

Ginseng: May improve mood and sleep quality.

3. Acupuncture:

Benefits: This ancient Chinese practice involves inserting fine needles into specific points on the body. It has been shown to reduce hot flashes, improve mood, and enhance sleep.

4. Mind-Body Practices:

Yoga and Tai Chi: These practices promote relaxation, improve flexibility, and reduce stress. They can also alleviate symptoms like hot flashes and joint pain.

Meditation and Mindfulness: Regular meditation can help manage anxiety, improve mood, and enhance overall mental well-being.

Tip: Natural and alternative therapies offer a holistic approach to managing menopausal symptoms. While results can vary, many women find these treatments beneficial. Always consult with a healthcare provider before starting any new supplement or therapy to ensure it is safe and appropriate for you.

Lifestyle Changes

Adopting healthy lifestyle changes can profoundly impact your experience during perimenopause and menopause. Here are some strategies to consider:

1. Nutrition:

Balanced Diet: Focus on a diet rich in fruits, vegetables, whole grains, lean proteins, and healthy fats. These foods provide essential nutrients that support overall health.

Calcium and Vitamin D: Essential for bone health, especially as estrogen levels decline. Include dairy products, leafy greens, and fortified foods in your diet, and consider supplements if necessary.

Hydration: Staying well-hydrated can help manage symptoms like hot flashes and support overall health.

2. Regular Exercise:

Cardiovascular Exercise: Activities like walking, swimming, and cycling improve heart health, boost mood, and help maintain a healthy weight.

Strength Training: Helps maintain muscle mass, supports bone health, and boosts metabolism.

Flexibility and Balance Exercises: Yoga and stretching improve flexibility and balance, reducing the risk of falls and injuries.

3. Sleep Hygiene:

Consistent Sleep Schedule: Go to bed and wake up at the same time every day to regulate your sleep cycle.

Relaxing Bedtime Routine: Activities like reading, taking a warm bath, or practicing relaxation techniques can help prepare your body for sleep.

Comfortable Sleep Environment: Keep your bedroom cool, dark, and quiet to promote restful sleep.

Tip: Small, consistent changes in your lifestyle can lead to significant improvements in your overall well-being. By prioritizing nutrition, exercise, and sleep, you can manage symptoms more effectively and enhance your quality of life during this transition.

Emotional and Mental Health Support

The emotional and psychological aspects of perimenopause and menopause are just as important as the physical symptoms. Addressing these areas can help you maintain a positive outlook and emotional resilience.

1. Support Networks:

Friends and Family: Sharing your experiences with loved ones can provide emotional support and reduce feelings of isolation.

Support Groups: Joining a menopause support group, either in-person or online, allows you to connect with others who are going through similar experiences.

2. Professional Support:

Therapists and Counselors: Professional counseling can help you navigate emotional challenges, manage stress, and develop coping strategies.

Cognitive-Behavioral Therapy (CBT): This form of therapy can be particularly effective in managing anxiety and depression associated with menopause.

3. Mindfulness and Relaxation Techniques:

Mindfulness Meditation: Practicing mindfulness can help you stay grounded, manage stress, and improve emotional well-being.

Breathing Exercises: Deep breathing exercises can reduce anxiety, promote relaxation, and improve sleep.

4. Creative Outlets:

Hobbies and Interests: Engaging in creative activities like painting, writing, or gardening can provide a sense of fulfillment and joy.

Physical Activities: Exercise not only benefits your physical health but also releases endorphins, which can improve mood and reduce stress.

Tip: Taking care of your emotional and mental health is essential during this transition. By seeking support, practicing mindfulness, and engaging in activities that bring you joy, you can maintain a positive outlook and emotional resilience.

Conclusion

Perimenopause and menopause are natural phases of life that bring about various changes and challenges. However, with the right approach, you can navigate these transitions with grace and optimism. Hormone therapy, natural and alternative treatments, lifestyle changes, and emotional and mental health support all play vital roles in enhancing your quality of life during this time.

Remember, every woman's experience is unique. What works for one person may not work for another, so it's essential to explore different options and find what works best for you. Stay informed, seek support when needed, and prioritize self-care. By embracing this journey with a positive mindset and proactive approach, you can thrive during perimenopause and menopause, enjoying a vibrant and fulfilling life.

Stay hopeful and encouraged—this is a time of transformation and new beginnings. With the right tools and support, you can navigate these changes confidently and emerge stronger and more resilient than ever.

6

Embracing the Journey with Hope

Perimenopause and menopause are transformative stages in a woman's life, marked by significant physical, emotional, and psychological changes. As we've explored throughout this book, understanding these changes and knowing how to manage them can make a world of difference in navigating this journey with confidence and hope.

Reflecting on My Journey

When I think back to my earliest memories of menopause, it was shrouded in mystery and misunderstanding. As a child, it was simply the "M" word—an enigmatic term used by older women and sometimes men to explain the unexplainable changes happening to women as they aged. Fast forward to today, and I find myself in that very place, but with a mission to demystify and challenge the outdated perceptions surrounding perimenopause and menopause.

My journey through perimenopause has been a blend of discovery and resilience. It wasn't until I found myself grappling with symptoms like thinning hair, unexplained rashes, persistent weight gain, and fluctuating moods that I truly began to understand the impact of this phase. Reflecting on my experiences, I realized that my body had been giving me signals long before I acknowledged them. From the highs and lows of adolescence to the hormonal whirlwind of pregnancy and postpartum periods, each stage was a precursor to the profound changes I would face in my 40s.

Insights and Encouragement

Throughout this book, we've delved into the science behind perimenopause and menopause, explored the symptoms, and discussed a variety of treatments and lifestyle adjustments. Here are some key insights to carry forward:

1. **Knowledge is Empowerment**: Understanding the biological processes and symptoms of perimenopause and menopause is the first step toward empowerment. It allows you to recognize what's happening in your body and seek appropriate treatments and support.
2. **Holistic Approaches Matter**: Combining medical treatments with natural and alternative therapies, lifestyle changes, and emotional support creates a comprehensive approach to managing symptoms. Each woman's journey is unique, and finding what works best for you is crucial.
3. **Emotional Health is Key**: The emotional and psychological aspects of menopause are significant. Building a strong support network, practicing mindfulness, and seeking professional help when needed are vital for maintaining

mental and emotional well-being.

4. **Self-Care is Non-Negotiable**: Prioritizing self-care through nutrition, exercise, sleep, and stress management can significantly enhance your quality of life. Small, consistent changes in these areas can lead to profound improvements in how you feel daily.

A Message of Hope

As I look back on my journey and the experiences shared in this book, I am filled with a sense of hope and resilience. The challenges of perimenopause and menopause are real, but so are the solutions and support available to us. It's important to remember that you are not alone in this journey. Millions of women worldwide are experiencing similar changes, and there is a wealth of knowledge and resources to help you navigate this phase with grace and confidence.

To my daughters, nieces, future granddaughters, and all the women who will walk this path, I want to leave you with this message: Embrace this time as an opportunity for growth and self-discovery. Celebrate your strength and resilience, and know that you have the power to shape your experience. By staying informed, seeking support, and prioritizing your well-being, you can transform this transition into a period of empowerment and renewal.

To the men in the lives of your wives, daughters, mothers, aunts, and woman partners or friends - approach this time with compassion and understanding. The woman in your life is even more confused than you are but taking the step to understand by reading this book is one way to support them. It's an emotional time so patience and care should be an utmost objective.

Take a deep breath, hold your head high, and step forward into this new era with hope and determination. This is not an ending, but a new beginning—a time to redefine and rediscover yourself. With the right tools, knowledge, and support, you can navigate perimenopause and menopause with confidence, emerging stronger and more vibrant than ever before.

Remember, this journey is yours to embrace, and every step you take is a testament to your incredible strength and resilience. Here's to a future filled with hope, health, and happiness.

7

Resources and References

Further Reading

The Galveston Diet: The Doctor-Developed, Patient-Proven Plan to Burn Fat and Tame Your Hormonal Symptoms - Mary Claire Haver MD **ISBN-10** ⊠ : ⊠ 0593578899

The Menopause Brain: New Science Empowers Women to Navigate the Pivotal Transition with Knowledge and Confidence - Lisa Mosconi PhD **ISBN-10** ⊠ : ⊠ 0593541243

The New Menopause: Navigating Your Path Through Hormonal Change with Purpose, Power, and Facts - Mary Claire Haver MD **ISBN-10** ⊠ : ⊠ 059379625X

It's Not Hysteria: Everything You Need to Know About Your Reproductive Health (but Were Never Told) Dr. Karen Tang ISBN-10 ⊠ : ⊠ 1250894158